I0472334

Cupping Therapy
for
asthmatic children

With
A summary of research thesis results

Dr. Tamer Shaban
2019

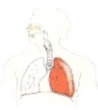

DR.TAMER SHABAN

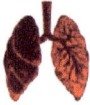

Copyright

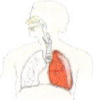

DR.TAMER SHABAN

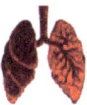

Disclaimer

Although the author and publisher have made every effort to ensure that the information in this book was correct at press time, the author and publisher do not assume and hereby disclaim any liability to any party for any loss, damage, or disruption caused by errors or omissions, whether such errors or omissions result from negligence, accident, or any other cause..

All information in this publication is for educational and information purposes only. Please consult your own physician for diagnosis or treatment of any health-related problems. The publisher and author are not responsible for any specific health or allergy needs that may require medical supervision and are not liable for any damages or negative consequences from any treatment, action, application or preparation, to any person reading or following the information in this book.

The Information on This publication does not dispense medical or professional advice, nor do they prescribe any treatment or strategy that should be tested without the advice of a professional. This book is not intended as a substitute for the medical advice of physicians. The reader should regularly consult a physician in matters relating to his/her health and particularly with respect to any symptoms that may require diagnosis or medical attention.

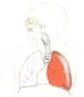

DR.TAMER SHABAN

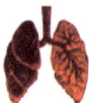

Preface

An academic professor once told me that cupping is lacking scientific evidence. He added that he did not find any clinical trials in the field of cupping therapy. This was fourteen years ago. From this date, I began my research journey to find, evaluate and develop this evidence.

I conducted my first clinical trial as a part of my master degree in child health between 2008 and 2010. There were also a plenty of clinical trials conducted in the past twelve years.

The first aim of this small book is to give the reader a brief introduction to the topic which includes: asthma, complementary medicine and cupping.
This brief introduction is updated by the recent information regarding this topic. The introduction is not a part of the thesis. Then, It gives a brief summary of the thesis which was discussed in 2010. The summary is organized and mixed with many new illustrations to make the topic easier for understanding.

The second aim of this small book is to help and motivate researchers in the field of integrative medicine to conduct new large scale randomized trials to provide scientific evidence regarding the safety and efficacy of cupping.
The third aim of this small book is to provide a hope for parents with asthmatic children which should be converted by policymakers to action plans and treatment programs.

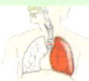

DR.TAMER SHABAN

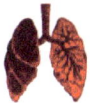

What is asthma?

Asthma is a chronic inflammation of the airways with reversible episodes of obstruction, caused by an increased reaction of the airways to various stimuli.
Airflow limitation in asthma is recurrent and caused by multiple causes which include: Bronchoconstriction, Airway edema, Airway hyperresponsiveness, and Airway remodeling. [1]

[1] National AE, Prevention P. Expert Panel Report 3 (EPR-3): guidelines for the diagnosis and management of asthma-summary report 2007. The Journal of allergy and clinical immunology. 2007 Nov;120(5 Suppl):S94.

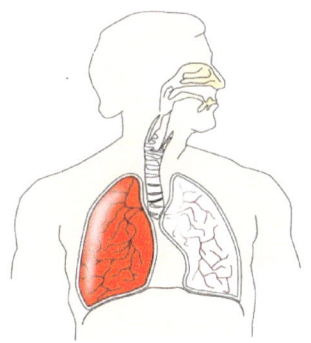

DR.TAMER SHABAN

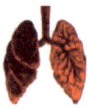

Burden of asthma

World Health Organization (WHO) reported that Asthma is the most common chronic disease among children.
And Asthma is under-diagnosed and under-treated.
It creates substantial burden to individuals and families and often restricts individuals' activities for a lifetime. [1]
According to the latest WHO estimates, 235 million people currently suffer from asthma, and there were 383 000 deaths due to asthma in 2015. [2].

[1] World Health Organization. Asthma-key facts . 2008.
[2]World Health Organization. Asthma-key facts . 2017.

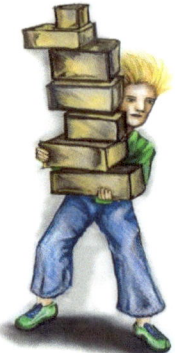
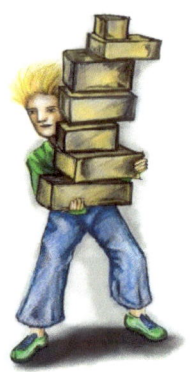

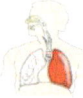

DR.TAMER SHABAN

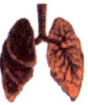

Complementary Medicine

Complementary medicine refers to a group of therapeutic and diagnostic disciplines that exist largely outside the conventional health care stream.
The name "complementary medicine" developed as the two systems began to be used alongside to complement each other . [1]

[1] Zollman Catherine, Andrew Vickers, ABC of complementary medicine: What is complementary medicine? BMJ 1999;319:693-696

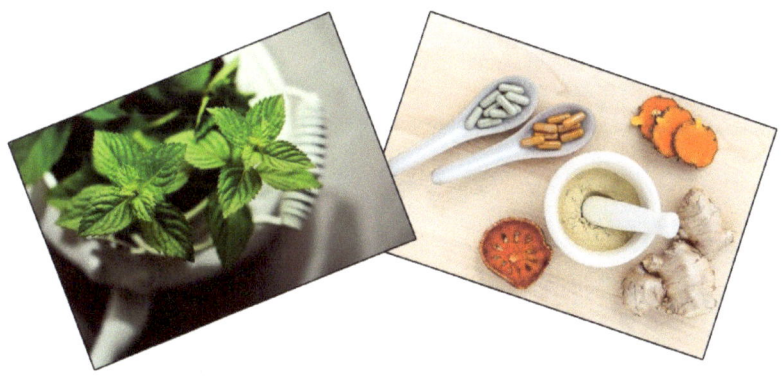

DR.TAMER SHABAN

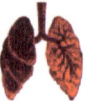

Complementary Medicine in medical schools

By 2003, 83% of US primary care medical school faculties had offered CAM courses within primary care curricula.

At least 40%of European Medical Schools offer courses involving CAM. Most medical schools in the UK offer CAM familiarization courses.

In Germany, CAM has become a required subject for all medical schools since 2003. CAM is also very popular in Switzerland. Two chairs for CAM were created upon popular demand at the Universities of Zürich (1994) and Bern (1995). In May 2009, a public vote was held in which 67% of the national population voted for the formal consideration of CAM. in the national constitution. Surveys assessing the status, prevalence, and diversity of CAM education in medical schools are available for the US, Canada, Australia, Japan, UK, Germany, and other countries. Collectively , these surveys indicate that CAM has established a significant presence in undergraduate medical curricula [1].

A Working Party of the Australian Medical Council Accreditation Committee in 1998 ascertained that all twelve medical schools in Australia and New Zealand provide at least some training in CAM as part of their degree [2].

[1] Nicolao Marie; Martin G Tauber; Florica Marian; Peter Heusser, Complementary medicine courses in Swiss medical schools: actual status and students' experiences, Swiss medical weekly : official journal of the Swiss Society of Infectious Diseases, the Swiss Society of Internal Medicine, the Swiss Society of Pneumology, SWISS MED WKLY2 010 ;140(3–4):44–51

[2]147. Weir Michael, What is complementary and alternative medicine, Bond University, Faculty of Law, Year 2005 Available online at: http://epublications.bond.edu.au/law pubs/65

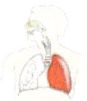

DR.TAMER SHABAN

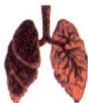

The prevalence of CAM practice by physicians

The prevalence of CAM practice is different depending on countries. For example, 51% of physicians in the United States practiced acupuncture, and vitamin therapy, herbal therapy, lifestyle diet, mineral therapy, and anti-oxidant therapy were frequently practiced by primary care physicians.

In the Netherlands, 51% of physicians practiced chiropractic therapy. Furthermore, in Germany, 78% of physicians practiced herbal medicine, and 45% homeopathy.

In Japan, CAM was practiced by 73% of doctors.

Japanese medical insurance system covers Kampo, and partly acupuncture, moxibustion, massage and spa therapy, while it does not cover other CAM therapies (1).

[1] 50.Fujiwara Kenji , Jiro Imanishi , Satoko Watanabe , Kotaro Ozasa , and Kumi Sakurada, Changes in Attitudes of Japanese Doctors toward Complementary and Alternative Medicine —Comparison of Surveys in 1999 and 2005 in Kyoto. eCAM Advance Access published on May 21, 2009, DOI 10.1093/ecam/nep040.

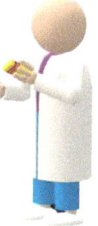

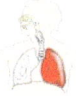

DR.TAMER SHABAN

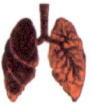

The Use of CAM Therapies by Children

Use of CAM for children with special health care needs is common. Its frequency and type are significantly associated with the child's condition and prognosis. [1]

Children with chronic illnesses are three times more likely to use CAM than a healthy population. [2]

Children who use CAM are more likely to be seeing their pediatrician for an illness, take medication on a regular basis, and have ongoing medical problems. [3]

[1] Sanders Heather, Davis Melinda F., Duncan Burris, Meaney F. John, Haynes, Julie Barton, Leslie L. Use of Complementary and Alternative Medical Therapies Among Children With Special Health Care Needs in Southern Arizona. Pediatrics 2003 111: 584-587
[2]McCann L J, S J Newell, Survey of paediatric complementary and alternative medicine use in health and chronic illness.
Arch Dis Child 2006;91:173–174. doi: 10.1136/adc.2004.052514
[3]Pitetti R, Singh S, Hornak D, Garcia SE, Herr S. Complementary and alternative medicine use in children. Pediatr Emerg Care. 2001;17 (3):165 –169

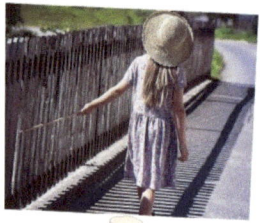
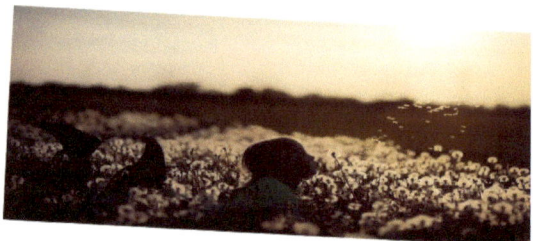
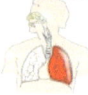

DR.TAMER SHABAN

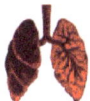

Prevalence and causes of use of CAM for asthma

The prevalence of using CAM therapies for asthma are varies, from 6% in adult to 65% in children (Partridge et al, 2008; Sidora-Arcoleo et al, 2007).

Some reasons cited for using CAM therapies include
1- Concern about the long-term effects of steroid use
2- Frustration that asthma does not resolve with conventional therapies;
3- Dissatisfaction with physician-patient interactions;
4- Belief that CAM is natural and, therefore, safe;
5- Desire to have autonomy in making health choices.
Several studies suggest that certain CAM therapies might improve the quality of life of children who have asthma. Promising data have emerged regarding some CAM treatments such as massage, and in patients having emotionally mediated asthma (Bukutu et al, 2008).

[1] Partridge M.R., M. Dockrell, N.M. Smith, The use of complementary medicines by those with asthma, Respiratory medicine 1 April 2003
(volume 97 issue 4 Pages 436-438 DOI: 10.1053/rmed.2002.1403)
[2]131. Sidora-Arcoleo Kimberly, H. Lorrie Yoos, Ann McMullen, Harriet Kitzman. Complementary and Alternative Medicine Use in Children with Asthma: Prevalence and Sociodemographic Profile of Users,
Journal of Asthma 2007 44:3, 169-175doi: 10.1136/adc.2004.052514
[3]Bukutu Cecilia, Christopher Le and Sunita Vohra, Asthma: A Review of Complementary and Alternative Therapies, Pediatr. Rev. 2008;29;e44-e49. DOI: 10.1542/pir.29-8-e44

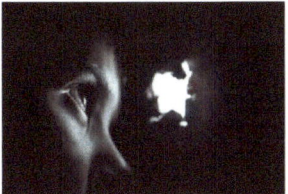

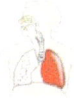

DR.TAMER SHABAN

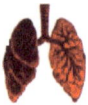

Cupping Therapy: Definition

Cupping Therapy is an old treatment method in which cups are applied to certain points or areas on the skin, either by heat or suction, to get health benefits. [1]

If puncturing or scarifications were made, the procedure is called wet cupping.

There are many types of cupping therapy (more than twenty types). we will mention later.

[1] Tamer Shaban. Cupping Therapy Encyclopedia - New Edition - 2018

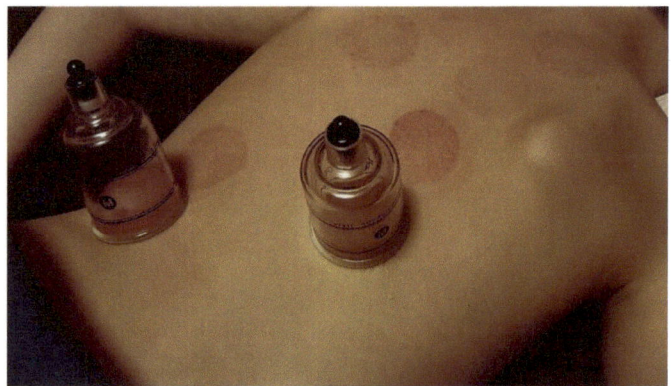

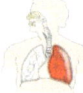

DR.TAMER SHABAN

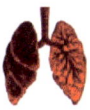

Cupping Therapy: History

Cupping Therapy in ancient China

Chinese medicine is one of the oldest medical systems in the world. TCM, or traditional Chinese medicine, uses many healing therapies and practices including acupuncture, herbal medicine, massage and Cupping Therapy. Cupping Therapy is a cornerstone in Chinese medicine. It was used successfully for thousands of years for the treatment of many illnesses. The oldest discovered book to mention cupping in China was written by Ge Hong (281-341 AD). Several centuries later, the classic book *Su Sen Liang Fang* recorded successful treatment of chronic cough and snake bites by Cupping Therapy.

Cupping Therapy in Ancient Egypt

Cupping Therapy was practiced in Egypt for thousands of years. The ancient medical book known as the Ebers papyrus was written in 1550 B.C.E, but is believed to have been rewritten from earlier texts, so the information it contains may be even older. The Ebers Papyrus contains about 110 pages, which when unrolled would be more than 20 meters long. The Ebers Papyrus mentions Cupping Therapy. Ancient Egyptians used wet cupping to remove foreign matter from the body. They prescribed Cupping Therapy for most diseases, and passed the practice on to the Greeks.

CUPPING THERAPY IN ARABIC AND ISLAMIC CULTURE

Prophet Mohammed (peace be upon him) treated by cupping (hijama in Arabic) and encouraged his fellows to use cupping (hijama) for the treatment of diseases. He said, "Cupping (hijama) is the best of your remedies." **Prophetic Medicine (Al-Tibb al-Nabawi):** This is one of the most famous Islamic books and was written by Ibn Qayyim al Jawziyya. It mentions Cupping Therapy as a medical practice.

Muhammad Ibn Zakaryia Al-Razi (865 - 925) was one of the best physicians and scientists in history; he was the first to differentiate smallpox from measles, and was described as the father of pediatrics. He benefited from Cupping Therapy in his treatment of many diseases.

Ibn sīnā (Avicenna) (980- 1037) was one of the most famous physicians in history, and author of the well-known *Book of Healing* and *The Canon of Medicine. The Canon of Medicine* was used as a textbook in the university of Montpellier as late as 1650. *The Canon of Medicine* stated that cupping was known to be effective on more than 30 different diseases.

GREEK HISTORY OF CUPPING

Hippocrates (460 BC -370 BC) was one of the greatest figures in the history of medicine and is called the father of western medicine. Hippocrates recommended using Cupping Therapy for a variety of diseases.

Galen (Galenus) (129 AD - 210 AD) was one of the most famous Greek physicians and medical researchers. Galen contributed to the fields of anatomy, physiology, pathology, pharmacology and neurology. Galen was a user of Cupping Therapy and he condemned Erasistratus, an Alexandrian physician, for not using cupping.

Then the art of Cupping Therapy was passed through the Alexandrians and Byzantines to Arab Muslims and Asians.

[1] Tamer Shaban. Cupping Therapy Encyclopedia - New Edition - 2018

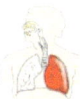

DR.TAMER SHABAN

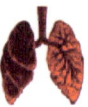

Cupping Therapy: Mechanisms of action

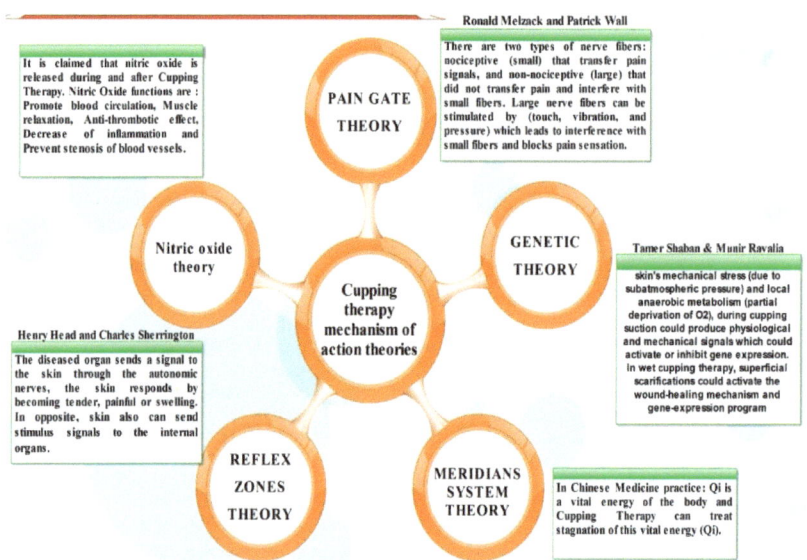

Ronald Melzack and Patrick Wall

PAIN GATE THEORY

There are two types of nerve fibers: nociceptive (small) that transfer pain signals, and non-nociceptive (large) that did not transfer pain and interfere with small fibers. Large nerve fibers can be stimulated by (touch, vibration, and pressure) which leads to interference with small fibers and blocks pain sensation.

It is claimed that nitric oxide is released during and after Cupping Therapy. Nitric Oxide functions are : Promote blood circulation, Muscle relaxation, Anti-thrombotic effect, Decrease of inflammation and Prevent stenosis of blood vessels.

Nitric oxide theory

GENETIC THEORY

Tamer Shaban & Munir Ravalia

skin's mechanical stress (due to subatmospheric pressure) and local anaerobic metabolism (partial deprivation of O2), during cupping suction could produce physiological and mechanical signals which could activate or inhibit gene expression. In wet cupping therapy, superficial scarifications could activate the wound-healing mechanism and gene-expression program

Cupping therapy mechanism of action theories

Henry Head and Charles Sherrington

The diseased organ sends a signal to the skin through the autonomic nerves, the skin responds by becoming tender, painful or swelling. In opposite, skin also can send stimulus signals to the internal organs.

REFLEX ZONES THEORY

MERIDIANS SYSTEM THEORY

In Chinese Medicine practice: Qi is a vital energy of the body and Cupping Therapy can treat stagnation of this vital energy (Qi).

[1] Tamer Shaban. Cupping Therapy Encyclopedia - New Edition - 2018

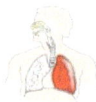

DR.TAMER SHABAN

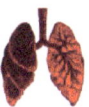

Cupping Therapy: Genetic Theory

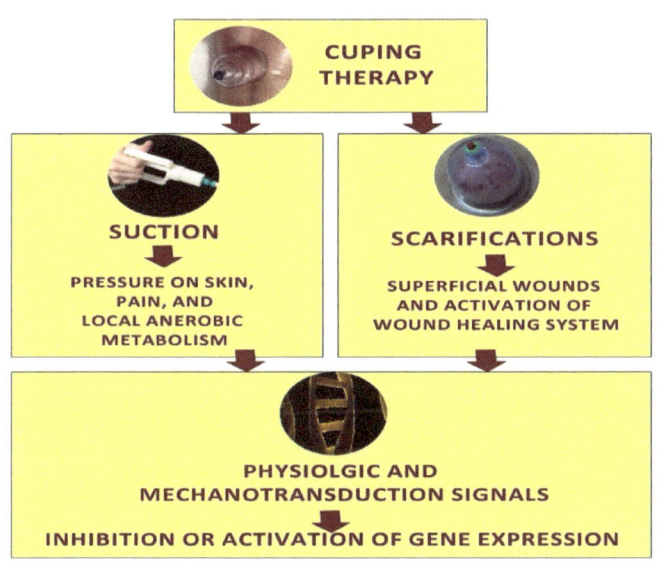

[1] Shaban T and Ravalia M. Genetic theory – a suggested cupping therapy mechanism of action [version 1; not peer reviewed]. F1000Research 2017, 6:1684 (slides)

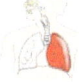

DR.TAMER SHABAN

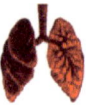

Cupping Therapy Effects

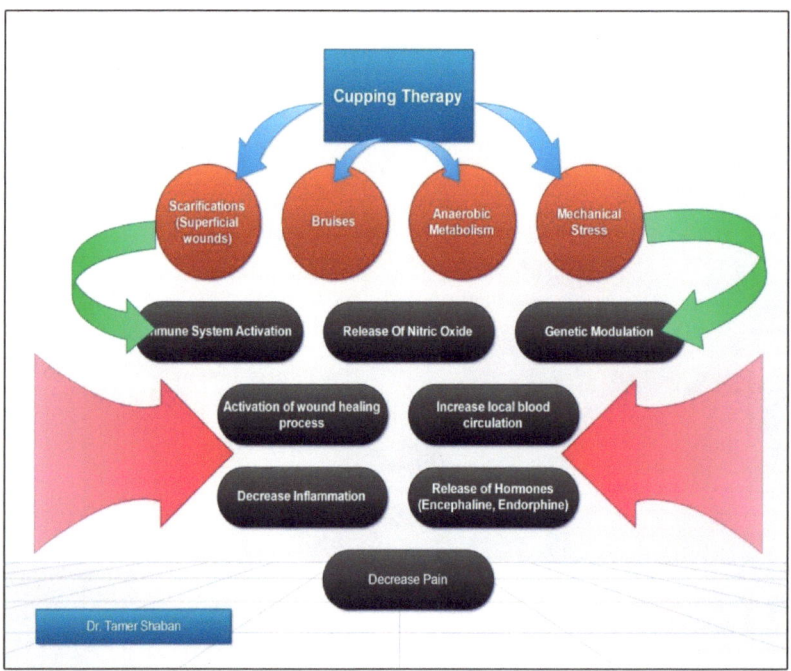

[1] Tamer Shaban - 2018

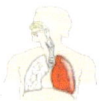

DR.TAMER SHABAN

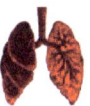

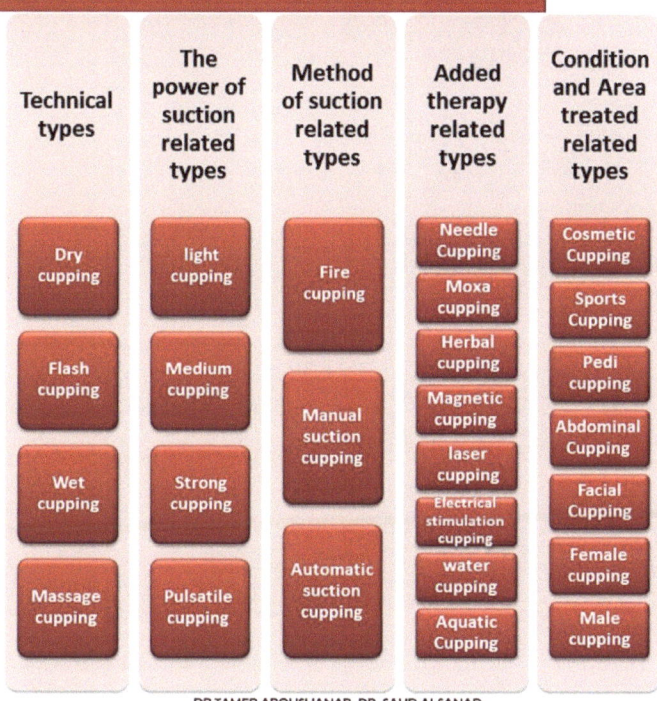

Classification of cupping therapy types

Technical types	The power of suction related types	Method of suction related types	Added therapy related types	Condition and Area treated related types
Dry cupping	light cupping	Fire cupping	Needle Cupping	Cosmetic Cupping
Flash cupping	Medium cupping		Moxa cupping	Sports Cupping
			Herbal cupping	Pedi cupping
		Manual suction cupping	Magnetic cupping	
Wet cupping	Strong cupping		laser cupping	Abdominal Cupping
			Electrical stimulation cupping	Facial Cupping
			water cupping	Female cupping
Massage cupping	Pulsatile cupping	Automatic suction cupping	Aquatic Cupping	Male cupping

DR.TAMER ABOUSHANAB, DR. SAUD ALSANAD

TO CITE:
ABOUSHANAB T, AND SAUD M. ALSANAD. CUPPING THERAPY: AN OVERVIEW FROM A MODERN MEDICINE PERSPECTIVE. JOURNAL OF ACUPUNCTURE AND MERIDIAN STUDIES, 2018-02 | JOURNAL-ARTICLE, DOI: 10.1016/J.JAMS.2018.02.001 .

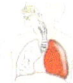

DR.TAMER SHABAN

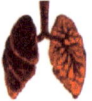

Cupping therapy types

Technical Types:
1- Dry cupping : A static type of cupping therapy. Cups are applied on selected skin points for up to 15 minutes.
2- Wet cupping: A static type of cupping. Superficial scarifications of the skin are performed either by surgical blade or by needle before applying cups to collect blood.
3- Massage cupping: A dynamic type of cupping therapy. Massage cupping is performed by applying a selected oil to the treatment area and applying a suitable cup by a mild to moderate suction,
Then, the practitioner should move the cup along the treatment area.
4- Flash cupping: A dynamic type of cupping therapy. Several medium to light pressure cupping are performed in a quick succession along the treatment area for stimulation

Power of suction:
5- Light cupping: When applying a light suction.
6- Medium cupping: When applying a moderate suction.
7- Strong cupping: When applying a strong suction.
8- Pulsatile cupping: A continuous changing pressure is applied by special device.

Method of suction:
9- Fire cupping: When fire is used as a method of suction.
10- Manual suction cupping: When manual suction pump, or self-suction cups are used.
11- Automatic cupping: When automatic cupping devices or electrical suction pumps are used.

Added therapy types:
12- Needle cupping: Acupuncture is performed then cups are applied over the needles.
13- Moxa cupping: Moxa is applied first, then the cups are applied over it.
14- Herbal cupping : Bamboo cups are usually used. Cups are boiled in a suitable herbal tincture then applied to the skin.
16- Magnetic cupping: The use of magnetic probes inside the cups.
17- Laser cupping: The use of laser probe inside the cup.
18- Electrical stimulation cupping: The cups are attached to electrical stimulation device. The patient receives cupping and electrical stimulation in the same time.
19- Water cupping: The use of warm water inside the cup.
20- Aquatic cupping: Cupping is performed under water. It is a combination of aquatic therapy and cupping therapy.

Condition and area treated types:
21- Cosmetic cupping: The use of cupping therapy for beauty purposes.
22- Sports cupping: The use of cupping therapy for the improvement of athletes' performance and rehabilitation
23- Pedi cupping: The use of various types of cupping on foot.
24- Facial cupping: The use of cupping on face for beauty or therapeutic reasons.
25- Abdominal cupping: The use of cupping on abdominal area for the treatment of obesity, reducing cellulite or treating digestive diseases.
26- Female cupping: The use of special cupping device for the breast enhancement.
27- Male cupping: The use of special cupping device (self-use) for support and enhancement of erection.

Dr. Tamer Shaban

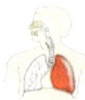

DR. TAMER SHABAN

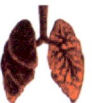

Flash Cupping

General information

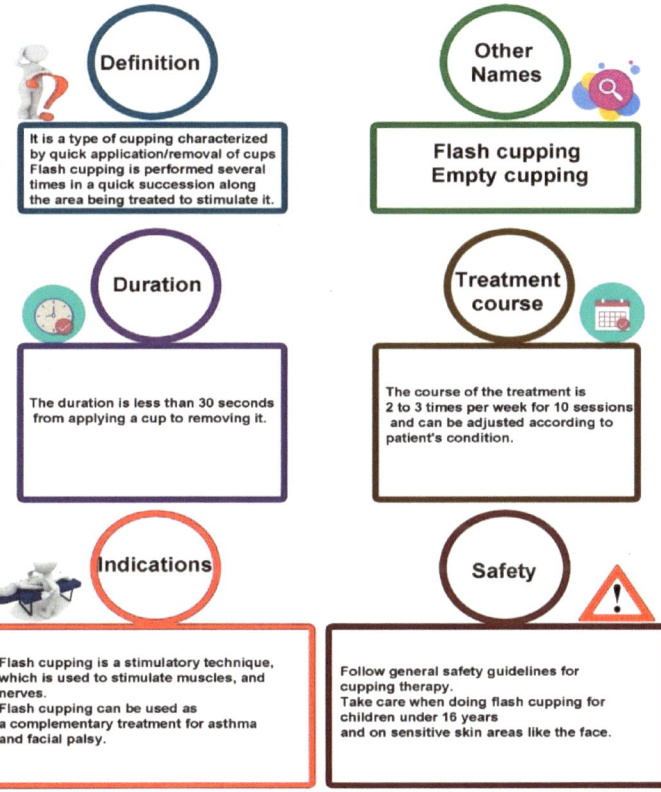

Definition

It is a type of cupping characterized by quick application/removal of cups Flash cupping is performed several times in a quick succession along the area being treated to stimulate it.

Other Names

Flash cupping
Empty cupping

Duration

The duration is less than 30 seconds from applying a cup to removing it.

Treatment course

The course of the treatment is 2 to 3 times per week for 10 sessions and can be adjusted according to patient's condition.

Indications

Flash cupping is a stimulatory technique, which is used to stimulate muscles, and nerves.
Flash cupping can be used as a complementary treatment for asthma and facial palsy.

Safety

Follow general safety guidelines for cupping therapy.
Take care when doing flash cupping for children under 16 years and on sensitive skin areas like the face.

DR.TAMER SHABAN

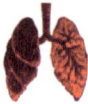

Classification of cupping therapy sets

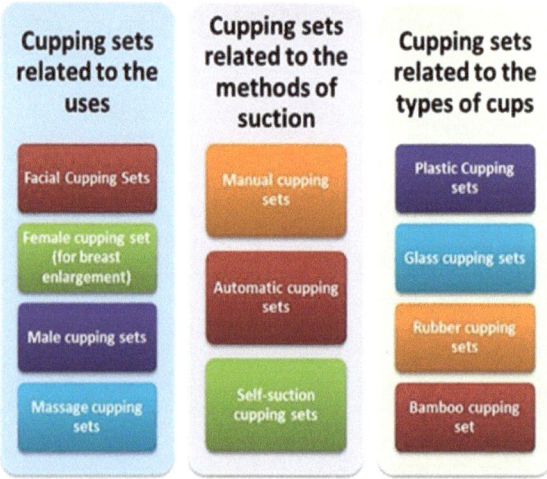

[1] Aboushanab, Tamer S., and Saud AlSanad. "Cupping therapy: an overview from a modern medicine perspective." Journal of acupuncture and meridian studies 11.3 (2018): 83-87.

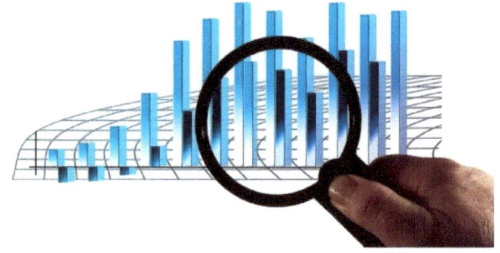

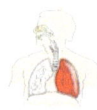

DR.TAMER SHABAN

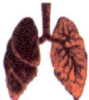

Cupping therapy indications

Cupping therapy can be used as:
1- A health promotion therapy
2-Therapeutic modality of variety of diseases.

It may be beneficial for pain-related conditions as reported by systematic reviews.

Common indications:
1- Low back pain [1]
2- Neck and shoulder pain [2]
3- Headache and migraine [3]
4- Knee pain [4]
5- Facial paralysis [5]

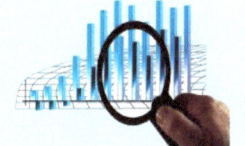

Cupping therapy could also be used in the treatment of other pain related conditions and musculo-skeletal diseases to complement other therapies, according to the patient's condition and doctor's advice.

[1] Kim, J. I., Kim, T. H., Lee, M. S., Kang, J. W., Kim, K. H., Choi, J. Y., ... & Choi, S. M. (2011). Evaluation of wet-cupping therapy for persistent non-specific low back pain: a randomised, waiting-list controlled, open-label, parallel-group pilot trial. Trials, 12(1), 146.
[2] Lauche, R., Cramer, H., Hohmann, C., Choi, K. E., Rampp, T., Saha, F. J., ... & Dobos, G. (2011). The effect of traditional cupping on pain and mechanical thresholds in patients with chronic nonspecific neck pain: a randomised controlled pilot study. Evidence-Based Complementary and Alternative Medicine, 2012.
[3] Ahmed, A. F., & Hssanien, M. M. R. (2010). Effect of cupping therapy in treating chronic headache and chronic back pain at Al heijamah clinic HMC. World Family Medicine Journal: Incorporating the Middle East Journal of Family Medicine, 8(3), 30-36.
[4] Teut, M., Kaiser, S., Ortiz, M., Roll, S., Binting, S., Willich, S. N., & Brinkhaus, B. (2012). Pulsatile dry cupping in patients with osteoarthritis of the knee—a randomized controlled exploratory trial. BMC complementary and a lternative medicine, 12(1), 184.
[5] Cao, H., & Liu, J. (2012). P04. 46. Cupping therapy for facial paralysis: a systematic review of randomized controlled trials. BMC Complementary and Alternative Medicine, 12(S1), P316.

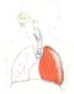

DR.TAMER SHABAN

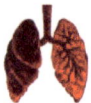

Cupping therapy indications

Indications of cupping :

6- Brachialgia [1]
7- Carpal tunnel syndrome [2]
8- Hypertension [3]
9- Diabetes Mellitus [4]
10- Rheumatoid arthritis [5]
11- Chronic Asthma [6]

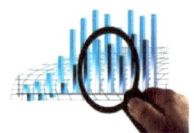

Cupping therapy could also be used in other diseases and illneses. Classification of cupping therapy indications is also developed and published. [7]

Local Cupping Therapy Indications	Systemic Cupping Therapy Indications
Neck Pain	Diabetes Mellitus
Knee pain	Hypertension
Low back pain	Fatigue
Muscle spasms	Rheumatoid Arthritis
Shoulder pain	Asthma
Headache and Migraine	Fibromyalgia

[1] Lüdtke, R., Albrecht, U., Stange, R., & Uehleke, B. (2006). Brachialgia paraesthetica nocturna can be relieved by "wet cupping"—Results of a randomised pilot study. Complementary therapies in medicine, 14(4), 247-253.
[2] Michalsen, A., Bock, S., Lüdtke, R., Rampp, T., Baecker, M., Bachmann, J., ... & Dobos, G. J. (2009). Effects of traditional cupping therapy in patients with carpal tunnel syndrome: a randomized controlled trial. The journal of pain, 10(6), 601-608.
[3] Lee, M. S., Choi, T. Y., Shin, B. C., Kim, J. I., & Nam, S. S. (2010). Cupping for hypertension: a systematic review. Clinical and Experimental Hypertension, 32(7), 423-425.
[4] Vakilinia, S. R., Bayat, D., & Asghari, M. (2016). Cupping therapy (Wet Cupping or Dry Cupping) for Diabetes Treatment. Iranian Journal of Medical Sciences, 41(3 Suppl), S37
[5] Ahmed, S. M., Madbouly, N. H., Maklad, S. S., & Abu-Shady, E. A. (2004). Immunomodulatory effects of blood letting cupping therapy in patients with rheumatoid arthritis. The Egyptian journal of immunology, 12(2), 39-51.
[6]al-Jawad, M. E. M. A., Saeed, A. M., Badawy, A. E., & Elfattah, N. M. M. A. (2011). Evaluation of wet cupping therapy (Cupping therapy) as an adjuvant therapy in the management of bronchial asthma. Indian Journal of, 5(4), 122.
[7] Aboushanab, Tamer S., and Saud AlSanad. "Cupping therapy: an overview from a modern medicine perspective." Journal of acupuncture and meridian studies 11.3 (2018): 83-87.

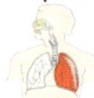

DR.TAMER SHABAN

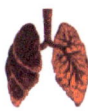

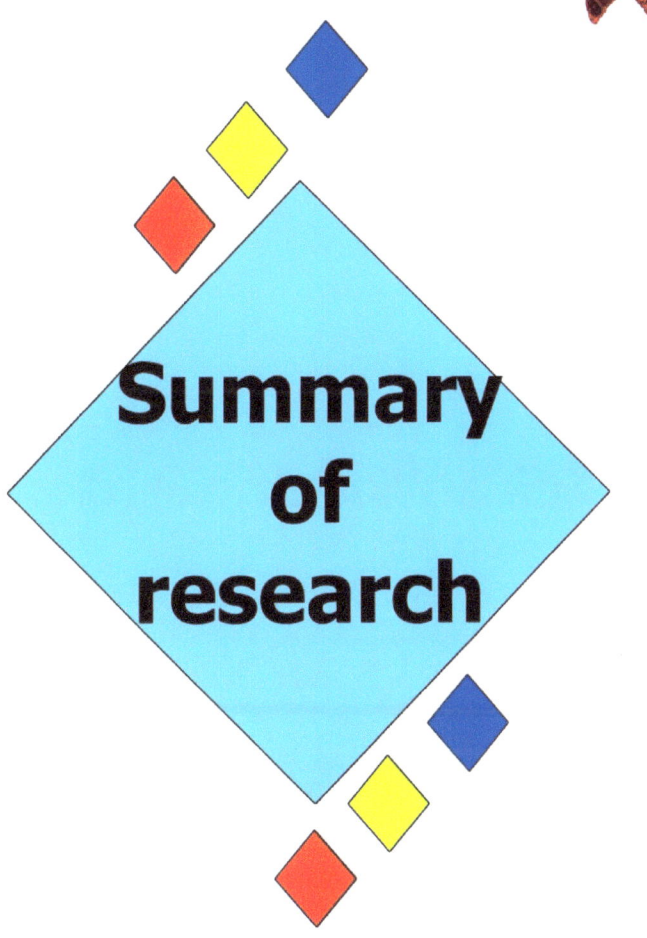

Summary of research

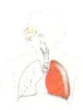

DR.TAMER SHABAN

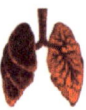

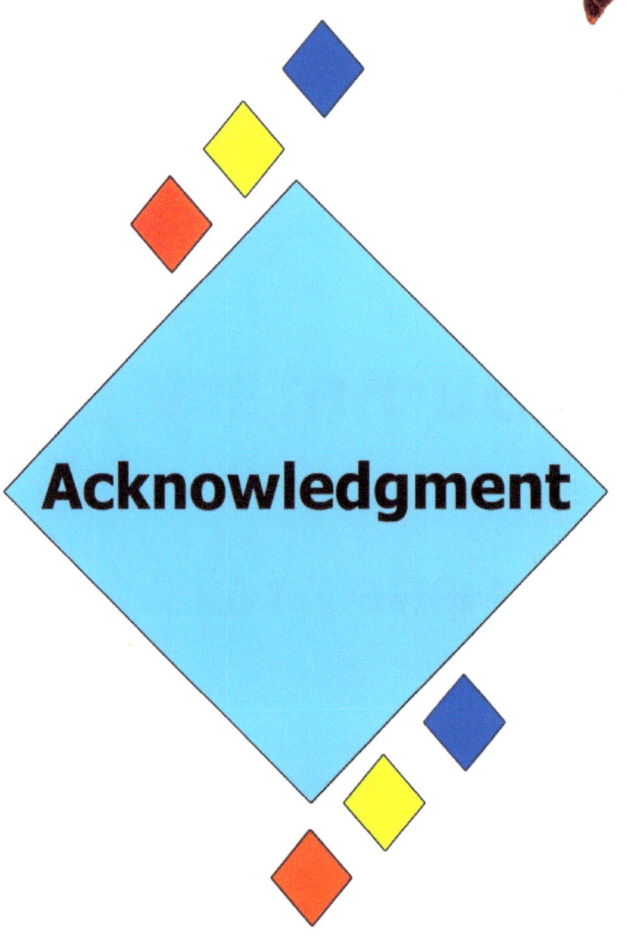

Acknowledgment

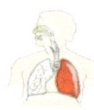

DR.TAMER SHABAN

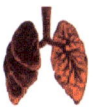

Acknowledgement

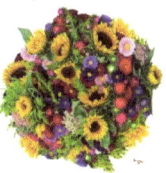

I am Greatly honored to express my great thanks to my supervisors:
Prof. Dr. Magdy Karam El-Deen Aly Daif, Head of Medical Studies Department Institute of Postgraduate Childhood Studies, Ain Shams University for his great support, encouragement and close attention throughout this work.

I am also greatly honored to express my great thanks to
Prof. Dr. Rehab Abd El kader Mahmoud, Professor in Medical Studies Department, Institute of Postgraduate Childhood Studies, Ain Shams University for her assistant, advice, valuable instructions and support in doing this work.

Finally, I am grateful to each one who helped me in this work, with special thanks to **Professor: Elizabeth F.Juniper;** the founder of pediatric Quality of Life Questionnaire for her special assistant by sending the translated Arabic version of the questionnaire and instructions, and with my great thanks to my parents and my wife.

Dr Tamer Shaban

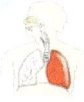

DR.TAMER SHABAN

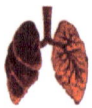

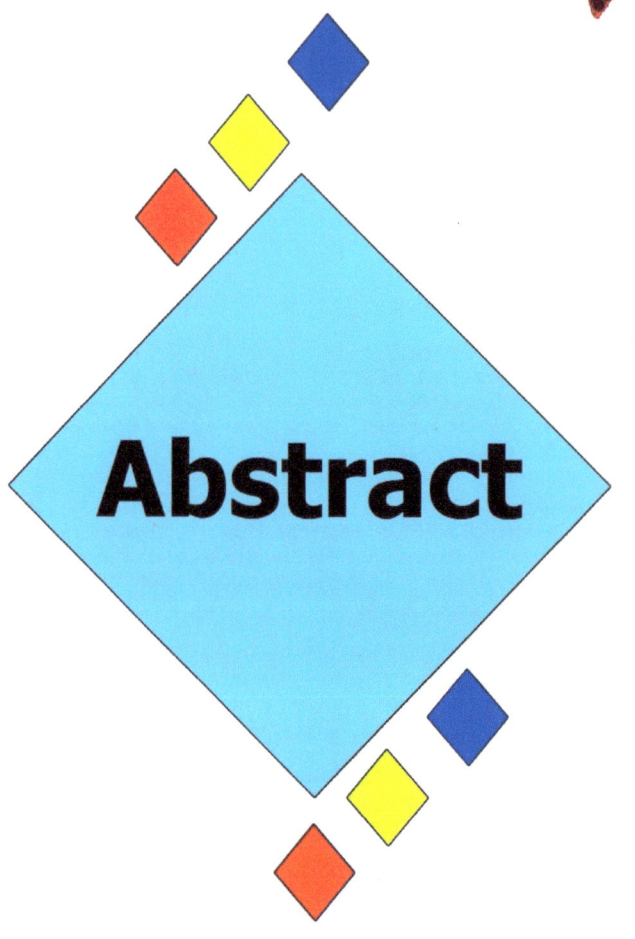

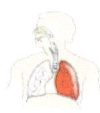

DR.TAMER SHABAN

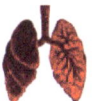

The Role of Cupping Therapy As A Complementary Therapy On The Pulmonary Functions And Quality Of Life Of Asthmatic Children

Master Thesis by Dr. Tamer Shaban

Abstract:

Aim:
The aim of this study was to evaluate the effectiveness of flash cupping therapy as a complementary therapy for the treatment of asthmatic children and adolescent in a randomized controlled trial.

Methods:
Sixty out-patients [8-15 years] with confirmed mild persistent asthma according to criteria of global strategy for asthma management and prevention were randomly assigned either to a treatment group [flash cupping therapy + standard asthma medications] [n=30] or a control group[standard asthma medications] [n=30]. Pediatric Quality of Life Questionnaire and Pulmonary functions [FEV1, FVC, FEV1/FVC Ratio, FEF 25%-75%] were measured before and after the treatment for both groups.

Results:
Improvement in all measured pulmonary function tests [FEV1, FVC, FEV1/FVC and FEF 25%- 75%], improvement in most of clinical symptoms, and improvement of pediatric quality of life questionnaire were found to be significantly higher in treatment group than in control group [p-value < 0.05].

Conclusion:
Cupping Therapy may be an effective complementary treatment for mild asthmatic children and has a significant improvement effect on the pulmonary functions and quality of life of asthmatic children. A large scale randomized control trial is recommended to confirm these results.

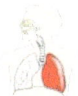

DR.TAMER SHABAN

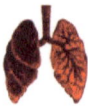

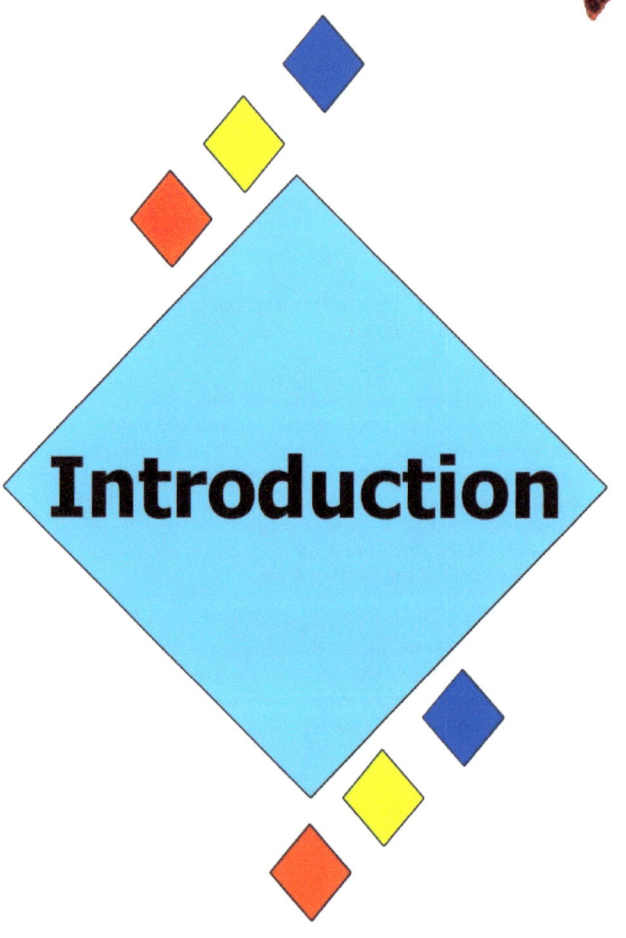

Introduction

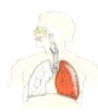

DR.TAMER SHABAN

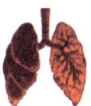

1. Introduction:

Asthma is a serious global public health problem. [1]
The burden of asthma in children is higher than recognized. [2]
The quarter of Egyptian asthmatic children were unable to
attend school regularly as a result of poor asthma control [2]
Asthma is the most common childhood chronic disease. [3]
Asthma is underdiagnosed, the prevalence of physician
diagnosis of asthma in Cairo was 9.4%. [4] The expression of
asthma is a complex process that depends on host factors
and environmental exposures which occurs during the
development of the immune system at a crucial time. [5]

Measurement of the quality of life is a new healthcare aspect
that can be represented as a marker in diagnosis and
estimation of the success of the total therapy. [6]
Evaluation of health-related quality of life should be
an essential aspect of clinical assessment of asthmatic
children to ensure the treatment benefits. [7]
quality of life was recognized as an important health
outcome measure in asthma. [8] The Pediatric Asthma Quality
 of Life Questionnaire [PAQLQ] is one of the most widely used
instruments for measuring health-related Quality of Life
in children with asthma. [9]

1. Paul O'Byrne. Global Strategy for Asthma Management and Prevention. preface. 2006.
2. Matthew Masoli, Denise Fabian, Shaun Holt, and Richard Beasley.Global Burden of Asthma . 104. 2006.
3. World Health Organization. Asthma-key facts . 2008.
4. Georgy, V., Fahim, H.I., El Gaafary, M., Walters, S. Prevalence and socioeconomic associations of asthma and allergic rhinitis in Cairo, Egypt .Eur Respir J 2006 0:
5. Expert Panel Report 3: Guidelines for the Diagnosis and Management of Asthma, Full Report 2007, National Heart, Lung, and Blood Institute, National Asthma Education and Prevention Program. U.S Department of Health and Human Services
6. Svetlana S.Pljaski, Dragoslav V.Djordjevi, Stojan S.Radi, and Borislav A.Kamenov. Asthma quality of life as a marker of disease severity and treatment evaluation in school children. Medicine and Biology 9[2], 175-180. 2002.
7. Elizabeth F.Juniper. How important is quality of life in pediatric asthma? Pediatr.Pulmonol , 17-21. 1997. Wiley-Liss, Inc.
8. Rutishauser, C., Sawyer, S.M., Bond, L., Coffey, C., Bowes, G. Development and validation of the Adolescent Asthma Quality of Life Questionnaire [AAQOL], Eur Respir J 2001 17: 52-58
9. Poachanukoon O, Visitsunthorn N, Leurmarnkul W, and Vichyanond P. Pediatric asthma quality of life questionnaire [PAQLQ]: Validation among asthmatic children in Thailand. Pediatr Allergy Immunol 17, 207-212. 2006.

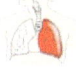

DR.TAMER SHABAN

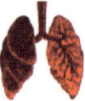

Complementary medicine

Complementary medicine includes all practices, therapies and ideas that are outside the stream of conventional medicine. [10] Complementary medicine is always used together with conventional medicine to complement each other. [11] Surveys assessing the status, prevalence, and diversity of Complementary and alternative medicine education in medical schools are available for the US, Canada, Australia, Japan, UK, Germany, and other countries. Collectively, these surveys reported that complementary and alternative medicine [CAM] had established a significant presence in undergraduate medical schools curricula. [12]

The prevalence of CAM practice is different depending on countries, 51% of physicians in the United States, 51% of physicians in Netherlands, 78% of physicians in Germany and 73% of physicians in Japan practiced a form of alternative and complementary medicine. [13]

The prevalence of using CAM therapies for asthma is varies, from 6% in adult to 65% in children. [14, 15]

10. Manheimer E, Berman B. Cochrane Complementary Medicine Field. About The Cochrane Collaboration [Fields] 2008, Issue 2. Art. No.: CE000052.
11. National Center for Complementary and Alternative Medicine. What Is CAM.
12. Marie Nicolao; Martin G Tauber; Florica Marian; Peter Heusser, Complementary medicine courses in Swiss medical schools: actual status and students' experiences, Swiss medical weekly : official journal of the Swiss Society of Infectious Diseases, the Swiss Society of Internal Medicine, the Swiss Society of Pneumology, SWISS MED WKLY2 010 ;140[3–4]:44–51
13. Kenji Fujiwara , Jiro Imanishi , Satoko Watanabe , Kotaro Ozasa , and Kumi Sakurada, Changes in Attitudes of Japanese Doctors toward Complementary and Alternative Medicine—Comparison of Surveys in 1999 and 2005 in Kyoto. eCAM Advance Access published on May 21, 2009, DOI 10.1093/ecam/nep040.
14. Partridge M.R., Dockrell M., Smith N.M., The use of complementary medicines by those with asthma, Respiratory medicine 1 April 2003 [volume 97 issue 4 Pages 436-438 DOI: 10.1053/rmed.2002.1403]
15. Kimberly Sidora-Arcoleo, H. Lorrie Yoos, Ann McMullen, Harriet Kitzman. Complementary and Alternative Medicine Use in Children with Asthma: Prevalence and Sociodemographic Profile of Users, Journal of Asthma 2007 44:3, 169-175

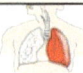

DR.TAMER SHABAN

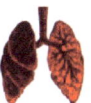

Cupping Therapy

Cupping Therapy is one of the oldest therapies. Cupping is a manual technique for breaking up localized congestion. [16] Ancient Egyptians were considered the first civilization practiced cupping therapy followed by ancient Chinese. The oldest recorded medical textbook [Ebers Papyrus] written in approximately 1550 BC in Egypt mentioned cupping. [17] Tham et al reported that Cupping is an effective alternative to needles in stimulating acupuncture points. Transmission of blood-borne diseases can be avoided as one of major advantages of dry and flash cupping, since skin is not penetrated. [18]

Empty cupping or flash cupping is a method of cupping that cups were applied rapidly and remain in place for a very short time less than 30 seconds. Flash cupping is the favorite cupping method for children. [19]

The main effects of cupping therapy in asthma management may be: improving the pulmonary functions in asthmatic children, normalization of blood gases in patients with persistent asthma, and prevention and treatment of early stage of external pathogenic invasion. [20, 21, 22]

16. Nicole Cutler, TCM Cupping and Massage: Part I, Institute for Integrative Healthcare Studies, October 08, 2008. http://www.integrative-healthcare.org/mt/archives/2008/10/cupping_for_mas-print.html
17. Kaleem Ullah and Ahmed Younis. An investigation into the effect of Cupping Therapy as a treatment for Anterior Knee Pain and its potential role in Health Promotion. TheInternet Journal of Alternative Medicine. 4[1]. 2007.
18. Tham LM, Lee HP, and Lu C. Cupping: From a biomechanical perspective. J Biomech 39[12]. 2005.
19. Ilkay Chirali, Cupping Therapy - Part Two, Chinese Medicine Times, Vol 2 Issue 2 - April 2007.
20. Hong Jiaxuan, Fu Mingli, Wang Xiaoyuan, and Gao Zhifeng. Effects of cupping therapy on pulmonary functions in asthmatic children. Journal of Traditional Chinese Medicine 26[1], 3-7. 2006.
21. Honora Lee Wolfe, The Effect of Puncturing the Network Vessels & Cupping on the Partial Pressure of Oxygen & Partial Pressure of Carbon Dioxide in Persistent Asthma, Blue Poppy Press, 2003.
22. Moses L and Wang BX. Study on cupping for diagnosis and treatment of early external pathogenic invasion. Zhongguo Zhen Jiu 25[9]. 2005.

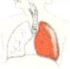

DR. TAMER SHABAN

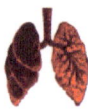

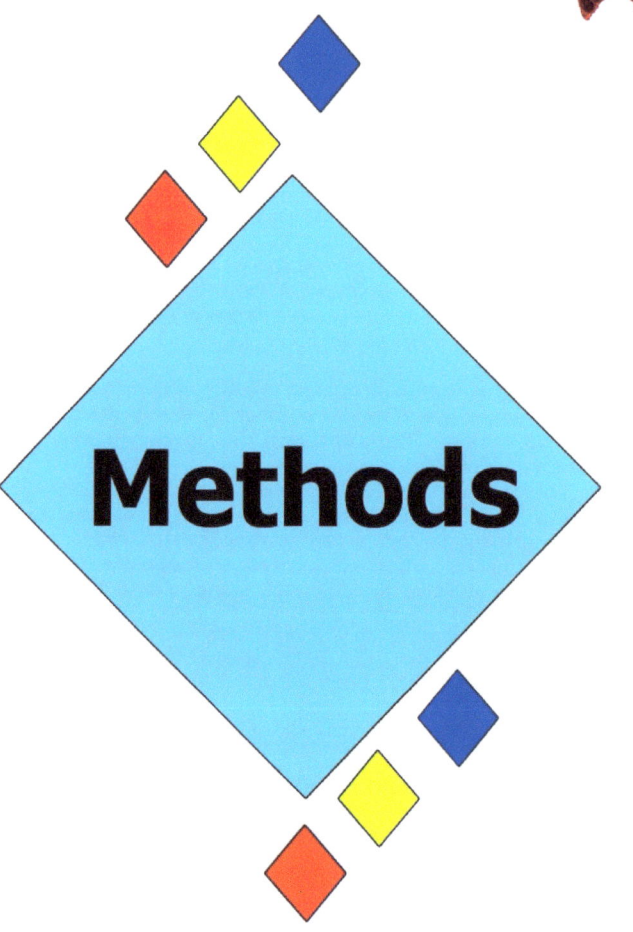

Methods

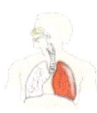

DR.TAMER SHABAN

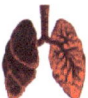

Patients and Methods

This study was designed as a randomized, controlled open trial.

The study protocol was reviewed and approved by the Committee of the medical department of Postgraduate Childhood Institute, Ain Shams University, Egypt.

Sixty out-patients [8-15 years] with confirmed mild persistent asthma according to criteria of global strategy for asthma management and prevention who fulfill the inclusion criteria were randomly assigned either to a treatment group [flash cupping therapy + drug treatment] [n=30] or a control group[drug treatment] [n=30] for comparative purpose.

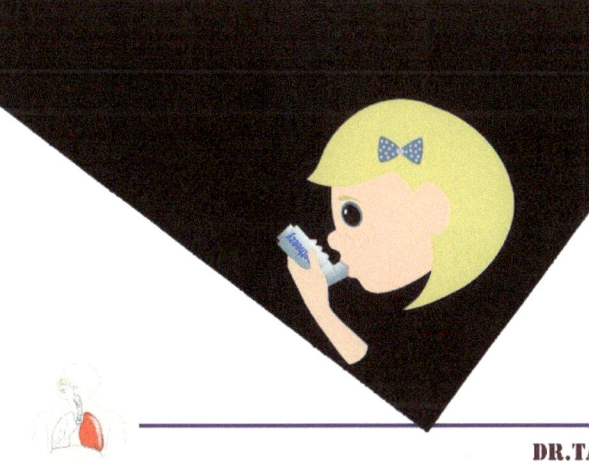

DR.TAMER SHABAN

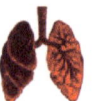

Inclusion and exclusion Criteria

Children between 7-16 years were eligible for enrollment to be suitable for performing pulmonary functions test, and who have confirmed diagnosis of mild persistent asthma according to global strategy for asthma management and prevention
[symptoms more than once a week but less than once a day, exacerbations may affect activity and sleep, nocturnal symptoms more than twice a month, FEV1 > 80%predicted, and FEV1 variability <20 - 30%]. Participants should between 15th percentile and 85th percentile according to Egyptian growth charts because overweight and obesity may affect pulmonary functions.
Children suffered from other chronic diseases such as [Diabetes, heart problems, and liver disease] or other asthma degrees were excluded.

Informed consent:
Written informed consent was obtained from each child's parent after explanation of the aim of the study and its benefit for their children and other children who have the same disease.
The steps of the study; the aims, the potential benefits and side effects were discussed with parents. They also informed about any abnormal results of procedure and tests performed.
There was no obligation for participation in the study.
Confidentiality of all data and tests results of all the study population were preserved. .
All parents of study participants gave their informed consent.

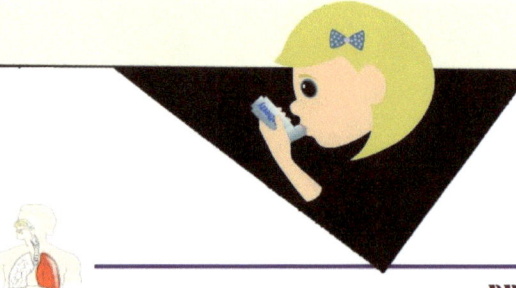

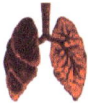

Study groups

Treatment group:

Thirty asthmatic children enrolled in the treatment group [8 Female and 22 Male] [8 to 15 years] with mean age of [10.73 ± 2]. The treatment group received standard asthma medications according to [Global strategy for asthma management and prevention and to flash cupping therapy

Control group:

Thirty asthmatic children enrolled in the control Include [7 Female and 23 Male] [8 to 15 years] with mean age of [10.6 ± 1.993]. Control group received standard asthma medications according to Global strategy for asthma management and prevention.

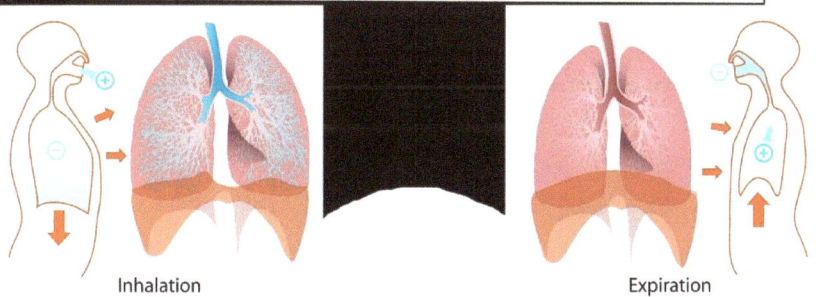

Inhalation   Expiration

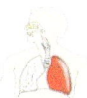

DR. TAMER SHABAN

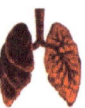

Outcome measures

Pulmonary functions:

It assessed the function of large and small airways before and after the course of treatment. The primary outcome measure was the improvement of various pulmonary functions. Pulmonary Functions included: FEV1,FVC,FEV1/FVC ratio,FEF25-75%.

Pediatric Asthma Quality of life Questionnaires [PAQLQ]:

[PAQLQ] is obtained before and after treatment. PAQLQ consists of 23 questions [items] divided into three categories [domains]: activity limitations [five questions], symptoms [10 questions] and emotional function [eight questions]. With regard to physical activities, patients themselves selected three of the activity limitation items. The answers were assessed by way of a seven-point scale, where one indicated maximum impairment and seven indicated no impairment. Improvement of PAQLQ was a second outcome measure.

Clinical parameters of asthma symptoms:

Improvement of episodic symptoms, cough, wheezing, chest tightness, and using of risk medications before and after cupping treatment was the third outcome measure.

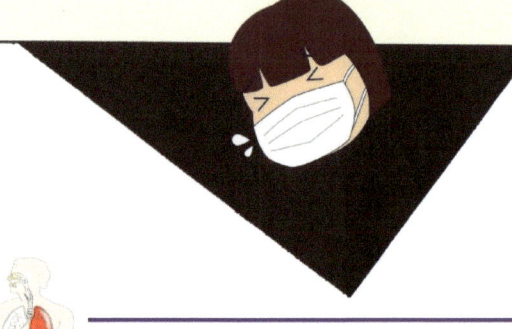

DR.TAMER SHABAN

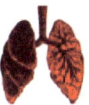

Intervention: Flash Cupping

Flash [Empty] Cupping Therapy:

Cupping therapy plastic sets was used including a hand suction pump, and single use disposable plastic medium size cups. Lubricant oil was used to facilitate application and removal of cups.

Empty [flash] cupping is performed according to procedure in table [1]. Selected points were on both sides of vertebral column, on chest wall muscles and sternum. The course of treatment was two times per week for five weeks. A total ten sessions were performed for every participant. The duration of every treatment was 15 minutes.

Flash cupping technique	
1	Hand washing
2	Wear clean gloves
3	Finding points for flash cupping
4	Swab with 70% isopropyl alcohol
5	Put the lubricant oil
6	Do mild to moderate suction [one to three full suction with the hand pump according to age]
7	Rapidly and for less than 30 seconds apply and remove the cup and move to the next point
8	Begin with the back and repeat on chest
9	Clean the oil after the treatment

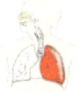

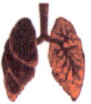

Flash Cupping Steps

1 Hand washing

2 Wear clean gloves

3 Finding points for flash cupping

4 Swab with 70% isopropyl alcohol

5 Put the lubricant oil

6 Do mild to moderate suction

7 Rapidly and for less than 30 seconds apply and remove the cup and move to the next point

8 Begin with the back and repeat on chest Clean the oil after the treatment

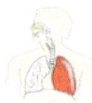

DR.TAMER SHABAN

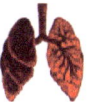

Flash Cupping Points

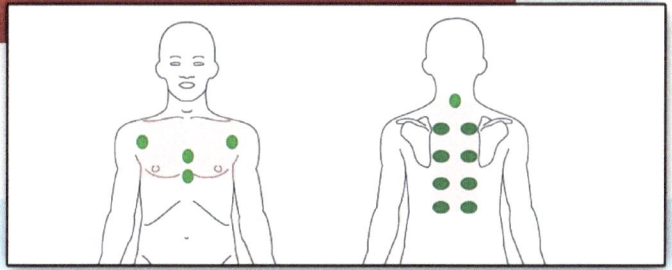

Flash cupping therapy at the back along both sides of vertebral column and at the level of 7Th cervical vertebra.
Then cupping is performed on the chest wall below the clavicle on both side and in the middle line on the sternum.

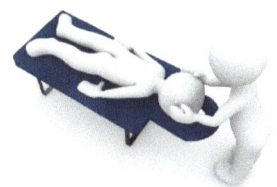

DR.TAMER SHABAN

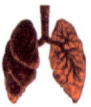

Statistical analysis

Statistical analysis was performed using the statistical software package SPSS version 13 [SPSS Inc].

Qualitative data as sex and disease characteristics were presented as numbers and percentages.

Quantitative data as pulmonary Functions and age were presented as means ± SD.
A probability value [p-value] less than 0.05 was considered statistically significant.

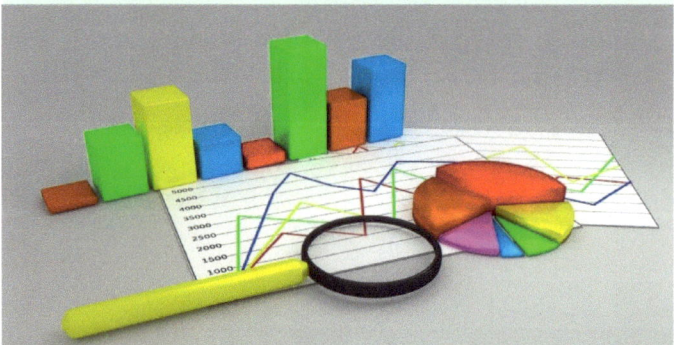

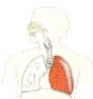

DR.TAMER SHABAN

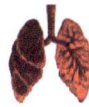
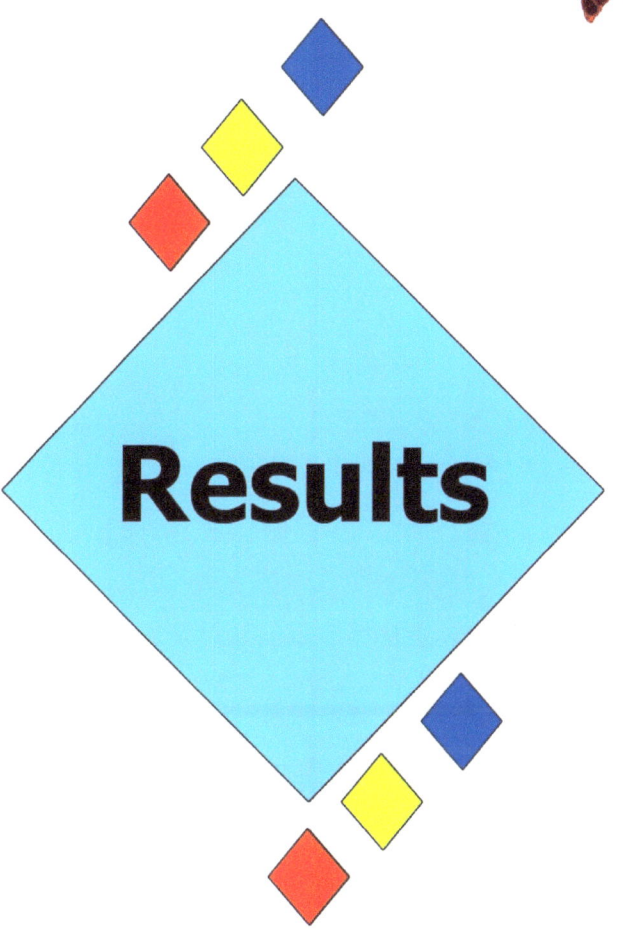

Results

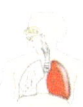

DR.TAMER SHABAN

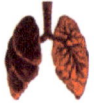

Results : Baseline

There is no significance of the baseline between study participants in both groups

		Treatment group [n = 30]	Control group [n = 30]	p-value
Age	Mean ± SD	10.73 ± 2.149	10.6 ± 1.993	[t-test] 0.8
	Range	8 – 15	8 – 15	
Sex	Male	22 [73.3%]	23 [76.7%]	[Fisher's [exact 1
	Female	8 [26.7%]	7 [23.3%]	
Height/Age	Mean ± SD	28.01 ± 6.07	28.46 ± 6.57	[t-test] 0.7
	Range	18-40	15-45	
Weight/Age	Mean ± SD	28.76 ± 5.79	29.06 ± 5.16	[t-test] 0.8
	Range	22 – 45	23 – 40	
Pulmonary functions				
FEV1	Mean ± SD	1.57 ± 0.30	1.43 ± 0.24	[t-test] 0.06*
	Range	1.06 – 2.39	1.08 – 1.99	
FVC	Mean ± SD	1.796 ± 0.343	1.65 ± 0.25	[t-test] 0.06*
	Range	1.17 – 2.58	1.21 – 2.29	
FEV1/FVC	Mean ± SD	87.03 ± 3.66	86.83 ± 3.61	[t-test] 0.84*
	Range	80.1 – 93.7	78.5 – 93.5	
FEF 25%-75%	Mean ± SD	1.9 ± 0.41	1.95 ± 0.36	[t-test] 0.661*
	Range	1.19 – 2.81	1.34 – 2.57	
PAQLQ				
PAQLQ	Mean ± SD	4.45 ± 0.74	3.94 – 0.55	[t-test] 0.075*
	Range	2.2 – 5.4	2.3 – 5.1	

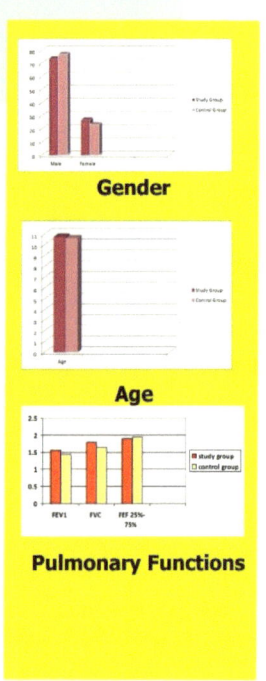

Gender

Age

Pulmonary Functions

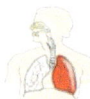

DR. TAMER SHABAN

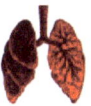

Results of outcome measures

**Treatment group
[Flash cupping therapy + standard asthma medications]
showed significant improvement of all measured pulmonary
functions, PAQLQ and most of symptoms than control group
[standard asthma medications]
as showed in Table**

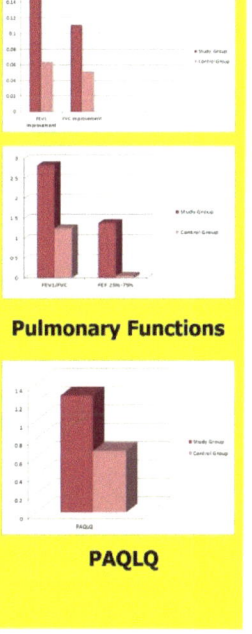

Pulmonary Functions

PAQLQ

		Study group [n = 30]	Control group [n = 30]	p-value
Pulmonary functions improvement				
FEV1 improvement	Mean ± SD	0.149 ± 0.078	0.069 ± 0.0759	[t-test] 0.000*
	Range	0.01 – 0.36	-0.1 – 0.17	
FVC improvement	Mean ± SD	0.11 ± 0.069	0.052 ± 0.083	[t-test] 0.004*
	Range	0.0 – 0.28	-0.14 – 0.15	
FEV1/FVC improvement	Mean ± SD	2.82 ± 2.62	1.25 ± 1.966	[t-test] 0.011*
	Range	-2.9 – 6.6	-2.4 – 7.9	
FEF 25%-75% improvement	Mean ± SD	1.38 ± 0.085	0.055 ± 0.083	[t-test] 0.000*
	Range	-0.02 – 0.32	-0.19 – 0.16	
PAQLQ improvement				
PAQLQ improvement	Mean ± SD	1.2733 ± 0.57532	0.6667 – 0.73828	[t-test] 0.001*
	Range	0.3 – 2.2	-0.5 – 2.1	

Pulmonary Functions and PAQLQ

DR.TAMER SHABAN

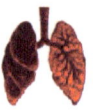

Results of outcome measures

Clinical Parameters

Treatment group
[Flash cupping therapy + standard asthma medications]
showed significant improvement of most of
symptoms and clinical parametes than control
group [standard asthma medications]
as showed in Table

symptom	N%	Treatment group			Control group			
		Before	After	Improvement	Before	After	Improvement	P-Value
Cough	N [%]	23 [76.7%]	2 [6.7%]	21[70%]	24 [80%]	12 [40%]	12 [40%]	0.02*
Wheezes	N [%]	21[70%]	3 [10%]	18[60%]	25 [83.3%]	16 [53.3]	9 [30%]	0.02*
Nocturnal Symptoms	N [%]	21[70%]	1 [3.3%]	20[66.7%]	23 [76.7%]	12 [40%]	11 [36.7%]	0.01*
Use of Risk Medication	N [%]	6 [20%]	0 [0%]	6[20%]	3 [10%]	1[3.3%]	2 [6.7%]	0.399

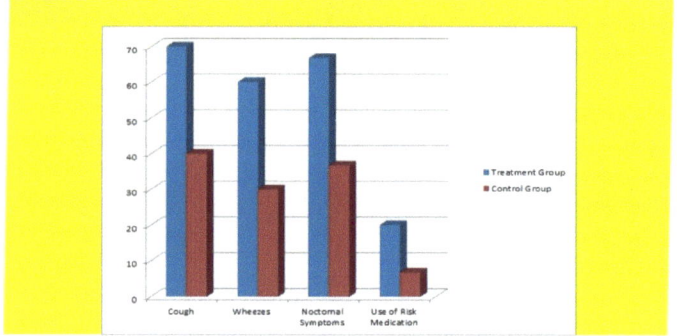

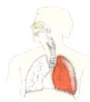

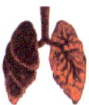

Safety

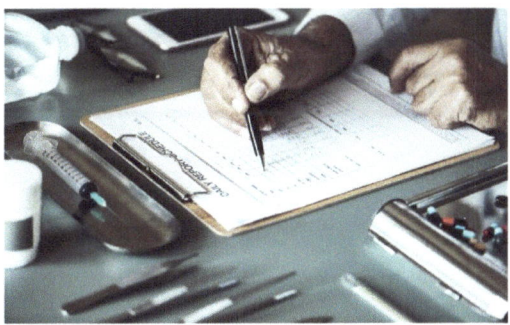

There were no serious adverse events in any of the study groups.
A mild to moderate discoloration was noticed in two of patients and disappeared next session .
The flash cupping procedure was tolerable.

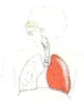

DR.TAMER SHABAN

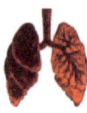

Discussion

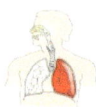

DR.TAMER SHABAN

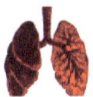

Discussion: Previous results

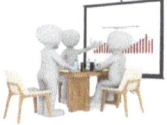

This study reported a significant improvement in pulmonary functions and clinical parameters including cough as a result of flash cupping therapy plus standard asthma medications medicine. Hong J. et al [2006], Liu X. [1996] and Zhang WP [2006] were in agreement with our results. Hong et al reported a significant improvement in most of pulmonary function values after cupping treatment of all mild asthma patients but no improvement of all severe asthma patients. [20, 21, 22] Liu X. [1996] reported the effectiveness of cupping therapy on back to treat children cough. [23] Zhang WP reported significant improvement of clinical symptoms and pulmonary functions in the treatment group [acupuncture + anti asthmatic agents] than control group [anti asthmatic agents]. [24]

20. Hong Jiaxuan, Fu Mingli, Wang Xiaoyuan, and Gao Zhifeng. Effects of cupping therapy on pulmonary functions in asthmatic children. Journal of Traditional Chinese Medicine 26[1], 3-7. 2006.
21. Honora Lee Wolfe, The Effect of Puncturing the Network Vessels & Cupping on the Partial Pressure of Oxygen & Partial Pressure of Carbon Dioxide in Persistent Asthma, Blue Poppy Press, 2003.
22. Moses L and Wang BX. Study on cupping for diagnosis and treatment of early external pathogenic invasion. Zhongguo Zhen Jiu 25[9]. 2005.
23. Liu X., Treatment of cough in children by cupping on back, J Tradit Chin Med. 1996 Jun;16[2]:125.
24. Zhang WP. Effects of acupuncture on clinical symptoms and pulmonary function in the patient of bronchial asthma. Zhongguo Zhen Jiu 26[11]. 2006.

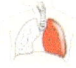

DR.TAMER SHABAN

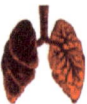

Discussion:
Cupping Mechanism in asthma

The mechanism of action of cupping therapy for asthma could be explained by some reported cupping physiological and mechanical effects. Cupping therapy may improve airway permeability, pulmonary hemodynamics, and the functional state of respiratory muscles. [25] Cupping therapy may have anti-inflammatory effect by an inhibitory effect on the uptake of neurotrophic factors. It may inhibit the synthesis and release of substance P in dorsal root ganglia. [26] Cupping had an immunomodulatory effect on allergic asthma.[27]
This study suggested a suitable and relatively safe method to help asthmatic children to improve the their quality of life. This technique could be learned by a family member to deliver flash cupping treatment. It may be a new tool for parents of asthmatic children.

25. Elena A.Shevchenko, adim Buevich, Elena E.Kalashnikova, Iraida G.Menshikova, Irina V.Skliar, and Marina Loevets. Acupuncture In The Treatment Of Patients With Chronic Obstructive Bronchitis: A Randomized Controlled Trial. Medical acupuncture Journal 16[3], 14-18. 2005.
26. Jun Tao Feng, Cheng Ping Hu, Xiao Zhao Li. Dorsal root ganglion: The target of acupuncture in the treatment of asthma. Advances In Therapy journal, Volume 24, Issue 3, P 598-601. DOI - 10.1007/BF02848784
27. Stefanie Joos, Claus Schott, Hua Zou, Volker Daniel, Eike Martin. Immunomodulatory Effects of Acupuncture in the Treatment of Allergic Asthma: A Randomized Controlled Study. The Journal of Alternative and Complementary Medicine. December 2000, 6 [6]: 519-525. doi:10.1089/acm.2000.6.519.

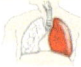

DR.TAMER SHABAN

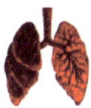

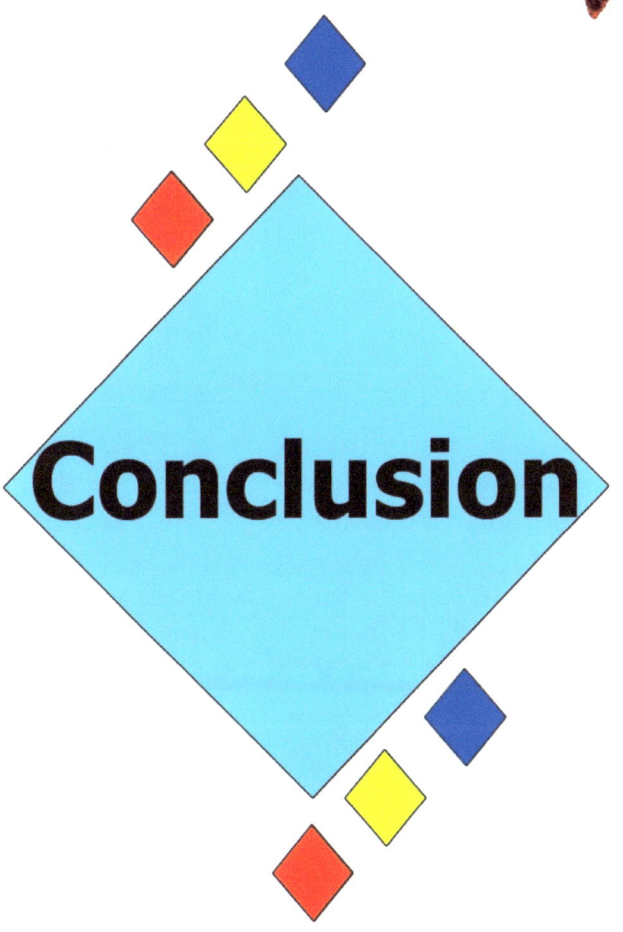

Conclusion

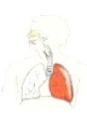

DR.TAMER SHABAN

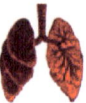

Conclusion

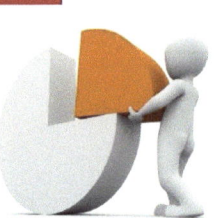

Flash cupping therapy may be an effective complementary treatment for mild asthmatic children;
it may improve pulmonary functions, symptoms and quality of life in combination with conventional anti asthmatic medicine. Largescale randomized clinical trials are recommended to confirm these results.

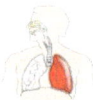

DR.TAMER SHABAN

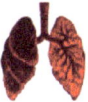

Recommendations

The author recommended the following:

1- Conducting a large scale clinical trial to confirm the results of the previous trials regarding the safety and eficacy of cupping therapy as a complemeentary treatment option for asthmatics.

2- Planning and developing of a self-care training program for the parents of asthmatic children which include training on flash cupping method, safety issues, and health education for asthma. So, The parents can provide a safe method that complement the modern medicine treatment.

3- Developing and implementing a complementary medicine course in all medical schools which gives an orientation, and essential knoweldge regarding safety and efficacy of complementary and traditional medicine modalities.

DR.TAMER SHABAN

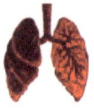

The author

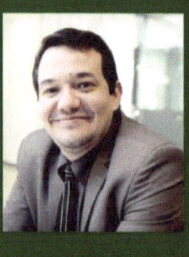

Dr. Tamer Shaban

Physician
Bachlore of medicine and surgery
Master of child health and nutrition

The author published three books in the field of cupping therapy. The most recent one is "Cuping therapy encyclopedia - new edition".

Contact:
tamer.shaban@gmail.com

Thank you for your time.

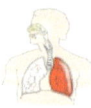

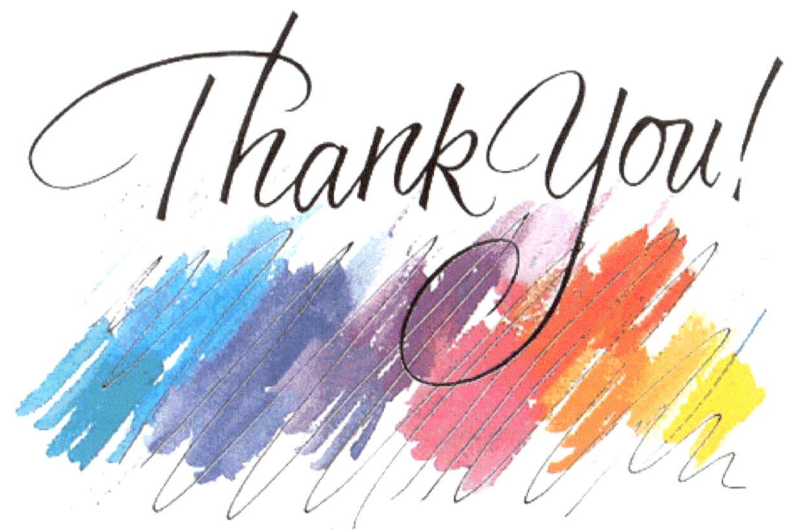